Created by <u>BabyDreamers.net</u>

Free Book Offer:

Get How to be a Super Mom For Free

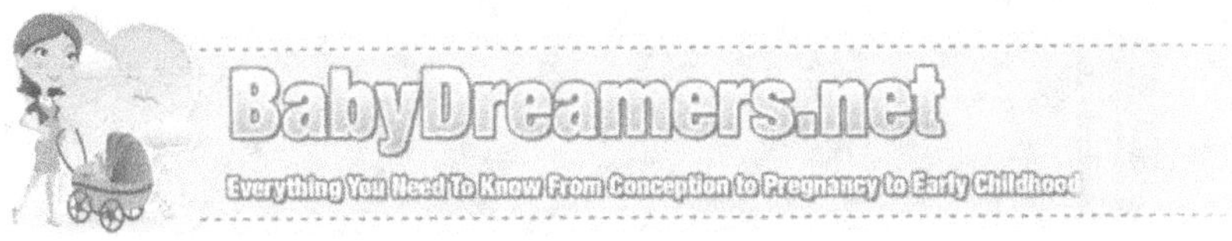

A Short Read is a type of book that is designed to be read in one quick sitting.

These no fluff books are perfect for people who want an overview about a subject in a short period of time.

Table of Contents

The Science Behind Getting Pregnant: Explained 8

Ovulation 11
Sperm Viability 12

Sperm Production 13
Sperm Health 14
Sperm Motility 16

Fertility Cycles 17

Follicular Phase 19
Ovulation Phase 20
Luteal Phase 21

Factors Affecting Fertility 22

Age 23
Health Conditions 24
Lifestyle Choices 25

Assisted Reproductive Technologies 26

In Vitro Fertilization (IVF) 28
Intrauterine Insemination (IUI) 29
Egg Freezing 31

Common Fertility Problems 33

Polycystic Ovary Syndrome (PCOS) 34

Endometriosis 36

Male Infertility 38

Optimizing Fertility 39

Healthy Lifestyle 41

Timing and Frequency 42

Stress Management 44

Frequently Asked Questions 45

Have Questions / Comments? 49

Get How To Be A Super Mom - 100% FREE 51

The Science Behind Getting Pregnant: Explained

The journey to parenthood is a fascinating and intricate process, guided by a multitude of scientific factors and processes. In this article, we will delve into the science behind getting pregnant, shedding light on key elements such as ovulation, sperm viability, and fertility cycles.

Ovulation plays a crucial role in the conception process. It is the release of a mature egg from the ovary, ready to be fertilized by sperm. Tracking and predicting fertile periods is essential for couples trying to conceive. By understanding the signs of ovulation, such as changes in cervical mucus and basal body temperature, couples can increase their chances of successful fertilization.

Another important factor to consider is sperm viability. Sperm, the male reproductive cells, have a limited lifespan. However, they can survive for several days within the female reproductive system, waiting for the opportune moment to fertilize an egg. This highlights the significance of timing intercourse during the fertile window, which is typically a few days before and after ovulation.

To better comprehend the science behind getting pregnant, it is crucial to explore the intricate processes involved in sperm production. In the male reproductive system, sperm is continuously produced in the testes. This ongoing production ensures a constant supply of healthy sperm, ready to embark on the journey towards fertilization.

Furthermore, the health of sperm plays a vital role in successful conception. Various factors can impact sperm quality, such as lifestyle choices, environmental factors, and underlying health conditions. Maintaining a healthy lifestyle, avoiding harmful substances like tobacco and excessive alcohol consumption, and managing stress levels can all contribute to optimal sperm health.

Sperm motility, or the ability of sperm to move effectively, is another crucial aspect of fertilization. Sperm must navigate through the female reproductive tract to reach the awaiting egg. Enhancing sperm motility can be achieved through lifestyle changes, such as regular exercise and a balanced diet, as well as avoiding excessive heat exposure.

The menstrual cycle and its impact on fertility cannot be overlooked. The menstrual cycle consists of three phases: the follicular phase, ovulation phase, and luteal phase. Each phase is characterized by specific hormonal changes and prepares the body for potential pregnancy. Understanding these phases can help individuals identify the most fertile period within their cycle.

The follicular phase marks the beginning of the menstrual cycle and is crucial for preparing the body for ovulation. During this phase, follicles in the ovaries mature and release hormones that stimulate the growth of the uterine lining, creating an optimal environment for a potential pregnancy.

Ovulation, the next phase, involves the release of a mature egg from the ovary. This is the prime time for fertilization to occur. Factors such as hormonal fluctuations, stress levels, and overall health can influence the timing and success of ovulation.

Following ovulation, the luteal phase begins. This phase is characterized by the production of progesterone, which prepares the uterus for possible implantation of a fertilized egg. If fertilization does not occur, the uterine lining sheds during menstruation, marking the start of a new cycle.

Various factors can impact fertility, and it is essential to understand their potential effects. Age is a significant factor, as fertility declines with age, particularly for women. Health conditions such as polycystic ovary syndrome (PCOS) or endometriosis can also affect fertility, requiring medical intervention or treatment. Lifestyle choices, including smoking, excessive alcohol consumption, and stress, can also have detrimental effects on fertility.

For individuals or couples struggling with infertility, assisted reproductive technologies offer hope. In vitro fertilization (IVF), intrauterine insemination (IUI), and egg freezing are among the options available. These technologies provide alternative paths to parenthood for those facing challenges in conceiving naturally.

Identifying and understanding common fertility problems is crucial in addressing obstacles to conception. Conditions such as polycystic ovary syndrome (PCOS) and endometriosis can affect fertility and require specialized treatment. Male infertility, caused by factors such as low sperm count or poor sperm motility, also poses challenges to conception.

To optimize fertility and increase the chances of successful conception, certain strategies can be employed. Maintaining a healthy lifestyle, including a balanced diet and regular exercise, can positively impact fertility. Timing intercourse during the fertile window and managing stress levels are also important considerations.

In conclusion, the science behind getting pregnant is a complex and fascinating field. Understanding the factors and processes involved, such as ovulation, sperm viability, and fertility cycles, can empower individuals and couples on their journey towards parenthood.

Ovulation

Ovulation plays a crucial role in the conception process. It is the release of a mature egg from the ovary, which then travels down the fallopian tube, ready to be fertilized by sperm. Understanding when ovulation occurs is essential for couples trying to conceive.

Tracking and predicting fertile periods can greatly increase the chances of successful conception. There are several methods to determine when ovulation is likely to occur. One common method is tracking changes in cervical mucus. As ovulation approaches, the cervical mucus becomes clear, slippery, and stretchy, resembling raw egg whites. This indicates the presence of fertile cervical mucus, which helps sperm to swim through the cervix and reach the egg.

Another method is monitoring basal body temperature (BBT). During ovulation, a woman's BBT rises slightly, indicating that ovulation has occurred. By tracking BBT over several months, patterns can emerge, helping to predict future ovulation. Ovulation predictor kits (OPKs) are also available, which detect the surge in luteinizing hormone (LH) that occurs just before ovulation. These kits can provide a more precise prediction of fertile periods.

Understanding ovulation and knowing how to track and predict fertile periods can significantly increase the chances of conceiving. By utilizing these methods, couples can optimize their timing and increase the likelihood of successful conception.

Sperm Viability

Sperm viability refers to the lifespan of sperm and plays a crucial role in the chances of successful fertilization. Understanding the lifespan of sperm is important for couples trying to conceive as it helps them determine the optimal timing for intercourse. On average, sperm can survive inside the female reproductive tract for up to 5 days. However, the chances of fertilization decrease significantly as the sperm ages. The highest chances of conception occur when intercourse takes place during the fertile window, which is typically a few days before and after ovulation. To increase the chances of fertilization, it is important to have intercourse regularly during this fertile period. Tracking ovulation can be done through various methods, such as monitoring basal body temperature, tracking cervical mucus changes, or using ovulation prediction kits. It is worth noting that the quality of sperm also affects its viability. Factors such as sperm count, motility, and morphology can impact the chances of successful fertilization. A healthy lifestyle, including a balanced diet, regular exercise, and avoiding smoking and excessive alcohol consumption, can contribute to improving sperm quality. In summary, understanding the lifespan of sperm and its impact on fertilization is crucial for couples trying to conceive. By tracking ovulation and optimizing sperm quality, couples can increase their chances of successful conception.

Sperm Production

Sperm production is a complex process that occurs in the male reproductive system. It plays a crucial role in fertility as healthy and viable sperm are necessary for successful conception. The process of sperm production, also known as spermatogenesis, begins in the testes.

Within the testes, specialized cells called spermatogonia undergo a series of divisions known as mitosis. This process results in the formation of spermatocytes, which then undergo meiosis to produce haploid cells called spermatids. These spermatids then mature and develop into fully functional sperm cells.

The entire process of sperm production takes approximately 64 to 72 days. It is influenced by various factors such as hormonal regulation, temperature, and overall health. Hormones like follicle-stimulating hormone (FSH) and luteinizing hormone (LH) play a crucial role in stimulating the production of sperm.

It's important to note that the quality and quantity of sperm produced can impact fertility. Factors such as age, lifestyle choices, and certain health conditions can affect sperm production. For example, advanced age in men can lead to a decline in sperm quality and quantity. Additionally, conditions like varicocele (enlarged veins in the scrotum) or infections can also impact sperm production.

To optimize sperm production and improve fertility, it is recommended to maintain a healthy lifestyle, including regular exercise, a balanced diet, and avoiding excessive alcohol consumption and smoking. It's also important to manage stress levels, as chronic stress can negatively affect sperm production.

In conclusion, understanding the process of sperm production and its impact on fertility is crucial for individuals and couples trying to conceive. By taking steps to optimize sperm production and overall reproductive health, the chances of successful conception can be increased.

Sperm Health

Sperm Health:

When it comes to conception, the health of sperm plays a crucial role. Healthy sperm increases the chances of successful fertilization and the creation of a healthy embryo. There are several factors that can affect sperm quality, and understanding these factors can help individuals and couples optimize their fertility.

One of the key factors that can impact sperm health is lifestyle choices. Certain habits such as smoking, excessive alcohol consumption, and drug use can have a negative effect on sperm quality. It is important to avoid these substances and adopt a healthy lifestyle to promote optimal sperm health.

Another factor that can affect sperm quality is age. Just like women, men also experience a decline in fertility as they get older. The quality and quantity of sperm may decrease, making it more difficult to achieve pregnancy. While age-related decline in male fertility may not be as significant as in women, it is still a factor to consider when trying to conceive.

In addition to lifestyle choices and age, other factors that can impact sperm health include certain health conditions and environmental factors. Conditions such as varicocele, infections, hormonal imbalances, and genetic disorders can affect sperm production and quality. Exposure to toxins, radiation, and excessive heat can also have a negative impact on sperm health.

To optimize sperm health, it is important to maintain a healthy lifestyle, including regular exercise, a balanced diet, and avoiding harmful substances. Regular exercise can improve blood circulation, which is essential for healthy sperm production. A diet rich in antioxidants, vitamins, and minerals can also support sperm health. Additionally, it is advisable to avoid exposure to toxins and excessive heat, such as tight underwear and hot baths.

It is important to note that while optimizing sperm health can increase the chances of conception, it may not guarantee pregnancy. If you are experiencing difficulties in conceiving, it is recommended to consult with a healthcare professional or a fertility specialist who can provide personalized advice and guidance.

Sperm Motility

Sperm Motility

Sperm motility plays a crucial role in the process of fertilization. It refers to the ability of sperm to move and swim effectively towards the egg for successful conception. Without adequate motility, sperm may struggle to reach the egg and fertilize it. Therefore, understanding and enhancing sperm motility can significantly increase the chances of successful fertilization.

There are several factors that can influence sperm motility. One of the key factors is the overall health and quality of the sperm. Sperm that are healthy and well-formed are more likely to have good motility. On the other hand, certain conditions or lifestyle choices can negatively impact sperm motility. For example, smoking, excessive alcohol consumption, and exposure to high levels of stress can all affect sperm health and reduce motility.

To improve sperm motility, it is important to adopt a healthy lifestyle. This includes maintaining a balanced diet rich in essential nutrients, vitamins, and minerals that support reproductive health. Regular exercise and staying hydrated are also beneficial for overall sperm health and motility.

In addition to lifestyle changes, there are certain supplements and medications that can help improve sperm motility. These may include antioxidants, such as vitamin C and vitamin E, which can protect sperm from oxidative stress and improve motility. It is important to consult with a healthcare professional before starting any new supplements or medications.

Furthermore, avoiding exposure to environmental toxins and reducing the use of electronic devices that emit electromagnetic radiation can also contribute to better sperm motility. It is advisable to wear loose-fitting underwear and avoid hot baths or saunas, as excessive heat can negatively affect sperm motility.

In conclusion, sperm motility is a crucial factor in successful fertilization. By understanding the role of sperm motility and taking steps to improve it, individuals and couples can enhance their chances of conceiving. Maintaining a healthy lifestyle, avoiding harmful habits, and seeking professional advice can all contribute to optimizing sperm motility and increasing the likelihood of successful conception.

Fertility Cycles

Fertility Cycles

The menstrual cycle plays a crucial role in a woman's fertility journey. Understanding how it works can greatly increase the chances of successful conception. The menstrual cycle typically lasts around 28 days, although it can vary from woman to woman. During this cycle, various hormonal changes occur, preparing the body for pregnancy.

One of the key phases of the menstrual cycle is the fertile window. This is the period of time when a woman is most likely to conceive. It usually occurs around the middle of the cycle, approximately 14 days before the start of the next menstrual period. During the fertile window, the ovaries release an egg, which can be fertilized by sperm. It is important to track this window to optimize the chances of conception.

Hormone fluctuations also play a crucial role in fertility cycles. The menstrual cycle is regulated by hormones such as estrogen and progesterone. These hormones help prepare the uterus for potential implantation of a fertilized egg. Hormone imbalances can disrupt the menstrual cycle and affect fertility. Tracking hormone levels and seeking medical advice if any irregularities are detected can be beneficial for couples trying to conceive.

It is worth noting that fertility cycles can vary from woman to woman. Factors such as stress, diet, and overall health can influence the regularity and length of the menstrual cycle. Keeping track of the menstrual cycle, noting any changes or irregularities, and seeking medical advice if necessary, can help individuals and couples better understand their fertility and increase their chances of successful conception.

Follicular Phase

The follicular phase is the first phase of the menstrual cycle and plays a crucial role in preparing the body for ovulation. It typically lasts for about 14 days, although this can vary from woman to woman. During this phase, the pituitary gland in the brain releases follicle-stimulating hormone (FSH), which stimulates the ovaries to produce follicles.

These follicles contain immature eggs and are located within the ovaries. As the follicles grow, they release estrogen, which helps thicken the uterine lining in preparation for a potential pregnancy. This increase in estrogen also signals the brain to decrease the production of FSH, allowing one dominant follicle to continue maturing.

As the follicular phase progresses, the dominant follicle releases increasing amounts of estrogen, which triggers a surge in luteinizing hormone (LH). This surge, also known as the LH surge, is a crucial event that indicates the impending release of an egg from the ovary. Ovulation typically occurs within 24-36 hours after the LH surge.

Understanding the follicular phase is essential for tracking and predicting fertile periods. By monitoring changes in cervical mucus, basal body temperature, and using ovulation predictor kits, women can identify when they are most likely to ovulate and optimize their chances of conception. It is during this phase that the body prepares for the release of an egg and sets the stage for potential fertilization and pregnancy.

Ovulation Phase

The ovulation phase is a crucial stage in the menstrual cycle where the ovary releases a mature egg. This process typically occurs around the midpoint of the cycle and is influenced by various factors. Understanding the ovulation phase and its intricacies can greatly enhance one's chances of conceiving.

During this phase, the pituitary gland in the brain produces a hormone called luteinizing hormone (LH), which triggers the release of the egg from the ovary. The surge in LH levels causes the dominant follicle in the ovary to rupture, allowing the egg to be released into the fallopian tube.

Several factors can influence the timing and occurrence of ovulation. The length of a woman's menstrual cycle plays a significant role, with ovulation typically occurring around 14 days before the start of the next period. However, this can vary from woman to woman, and tracking ovulation using methods like basal body temperature charting or ovulation predictor kits can provide more accurate predictions.

Other factors that can influence ovulation include hormonal imbalances, stress, and certain medical conditions. Hormonal imbalances, such as polycystic ovary syndrome (PCOS), can disrupt the regular release of eggs. Stress can also impact ovulation by affecting hormone levels and disrupting the delicate balance needed for successful conception.

It's important to note that not all women experience ovulation every month. Irregular ovulation or anovulation (lack of ovulation) can occur due to various reasons, including age, hormonal imbalances, or underlying health conditions. If you are struggling with irregular ovulation or suspect that you may not be ovulating regularly, it is advisable to consult with a healthcare professional for further evaluation and guidance.

Luteal Phase

The luteal phase is an essential part of the menstrual cycle that occurs after ovulation. It plays a crucial role in preparing the uterus for possible implantation of a fertilized egg. This phase typically lasts for about 10 to 16 days and is characterized by the presence of the hormone progesterone.

During the luteal phase, the ruptured follicle from which the egg was released transforms into a structure called the corpus luteum. The corpus luteum produces progesterone, which helps thicken the lining of the uterus, known as the endometrium. This thickened endometrium provides a nourishing environment for a fertilized egg to implant and develop into a pregnancy.

If fertilization does not occur, the corpus luteum gradually breaks down, leading to a decrease in progesterone levels. This decline in progesterone triggers the shedding of the uterine lining, resulting in menstruation and the start of a new menstrual cycle.

It is important to note that the length of the luteal phase can vary from woman to woman. A shorter luteal phase may indicate a potential issue with fertility, as it may not provide enough time for a fertilized egg to implant properly. In such cases, it is recommended to consult with a healthcare professional for further evaluation and guidance.

Factors Affecting Fertility

Factors Affecting Fertility

When it comes to fertility, there are several factors that can have a significant impact on a person's ability to conceive. Understanding these factors is crucial for individuals and couples who are trying to start a family. Let's explore some of the key factors that can affect fertility:

- **Age:** Age plays a crucial role in fertility, especially for women. As women get older, their fertility declines due to a decrease in the number and quality of eggs. It is important to keep in mind that fertility starts to decline significantly after the age of 35.
- **Health Conditions:** Certain health conditions can have a negative impact on fertility. Conditions such as polycystic ovary syndrome (PCOS) and endometriosis can affect the reproductive system and make it more difficult to conceive. It is important to seek medical

advice and treatment for any underlying health conditions that may be impacting fertility.

- **Lifestyle Choices:** Lifestyle choices can also influence fertility. Factors such as smoking, excessive alcohol consumption, and high levels of stress can all affect reproductive health. Making positive lifestyle choices, such as quitting smoking, reducing alcohol intake, and managing stress, can help improve fertility.

By understanding and addressing these factors, individuals and couples can take proactive steps to optimize their fertility and increase their chances of successful conception. It is important to consult with healthcare professionals and fertility specialists for personalized advice and guidance.

Age

As women age, their fertility naturally declines. This is due to several factors that affect the quality and quantity of eggs in the ovaries. Women are born with a finite number of eggs, and as they age, the number decreases while the quality diminishes. This decline in egg quality and quantity makes it increasingly difficult for women to conceive as they get older.

One of the main reasons for the decline in fertility with age is the decreased ovarian reserve. Ovarian reserve refers to the number of eggs a woman has remaining in her ovaries. As women age, the number of eggs decreases, and the remaining eggs may have genetic abnormalities or be less viable for fertilization.

Additionally, as women age, the hormonal balance in their bodies changes. The levels of hormones that regulate the menstrual cycle, such as follicle-stimulating hormone (FSH) and luteinizing hormone (LH), fluctuate. These hormonal changes can affect the timing of ovulation and the overall fertility of a woman.

It is important to note that while age has a significant impact on female fertility, it also affects male fertility. As men age, the quality and quantity of sperm may decline, making it more challenging for them to father a child.

Overall, age plays a crucial role in fertility, and it is essential for individuals and couples to be aware of the potential decline in fertility as they get older. Understanding the relationship between age and fertility can help individuals make informed decisions about family planning and seek appropriate medical assistance if needed.

Health Conditions

Health conditions can play a significant role in fertility, with certain conditions impacting a person's ability to conceive. Two common health conditions that can affect fertility are polycystic ovary syndrome (PCOS) and endometriosis.

Polycystic ovary syndrome (PCOS) is a hormonal disorder that affects women of reproductive age. It is characterized by the presence of multiple cysts on the ovaries and hormonal imbalances. PCOS can disrupt the regular ovulation process, making it difficult for eggs to mature and be released from the ovaries. This can result in irregular menstrual cycles and difficulties in conceiving. Additionally, PCOS is associated with insulin resistance, which can further impact fertility.

Endometriosis is a condition where the tissue that normally lines the uterus grows outside of it. This can cause inflammation, scarring, and the formation of adhesions, which can affect the function of the reproductive organs. Endometriosis can lead to pelvic pain, painful periods, and infertility. The abnormal tissue growth can block or damage the fallopian tubes, making it difficult for the egg to travel from the ovaries to the uterus for fertilization.

It is important for individuals with these health conditions to seek medical guidance and treatment options if they are trying to conceive. Fertility treatments and interventions may be available to help manage the impact of these health conditions on fertility.

Lifestyle Choices

When it comes to fertility, lifestyle choices can play a significant role in determining the chances of successful conception. Certain habits and behaviors can have a direct impact on reproductive health and fertility. Let's take a closer look at some lifestyle choices that can affect fertility:

- **Smoking:** Smoking has been shown to have detrimental effects on both male and female fertility. It can decrease sperm count and motility in men, while in women, it can lead to hormonal imbalances and damage to the eggs. Quitting smoking is crucial for those trying to conceive.

- **Alcohol Consumption:** Excessive alcohol consumption can disrupt hormone levels and impair reproductive function in both men and women. It is advisable to limit alcohol intake or avoid it altogether when trying to conceive.
- **Stress:** Chronic stress can interfere with the hormonal balance necessary for ovulation and sperm production. Finding healthy ways to manage stress, such as exercise, meditation, or therapy, can help improve fertility.

It's important to note that making positive changes in lifestyle choices can significantly enhance fertility and increase the chances of successful conception. By adopting a healthy lifestyle, individuals and couples can optimize their reproductive health and create the best possible environment for a baby to thrive.

Assisted Reproductive Technologies

Assisted Reproductive Technologies (ART) have revolutionized the field of fertility treatment, offering hope to individuals and couples struggling with infertility. These advanced techniques utilize medical interventions to assist in the process of conception and increase the chances of successful pregnancy. Let's explore some of the most commonly used ART options:

- **In Vitro Fertilization (IVF):** IVF is a widely known and highly successful ART method. It involves the retrieval of eggs from the woman's ovaries, which are then fertilized with sperm in a laboratory. The resulting embryos are then transferred back into the woman's uterus, where they have the potential to implant and develop into a pregnancy.
- **Intrauterine Insemination (IUI):** IUI is a less invasive ART procedure that involves the direct placement of prepared sperm into the woman's uterus during her fertile window. This method is often used when there are issues with sperm quality or cervical factors that may hinder natural conception.
- **Egg Freezing:** Egg freezing, also known as oocyte cryopreservation, is a technique that allows women to preserve their eggs for future use. This option is particularly beneficial for women who may face fertility challenges due to age, medical treatments, or personal circumstances.

These ART options provide a glimmer of hope for individuals or couples facing infertility. However, it is important to consult with a fertility specialist to determine the most suitable treatment plan based on individual circumstances. The advancements in assisted reproductive technologies have opened doors to parenthood for many, offering a ray of hope and the possibility of fulfilling the dream of having a child.

In Vitro Fertilization (IVF)

In Vitro Fertilization (IVF)

IVF, also known as in vitro fertilization, is a fertility treatment that has helped countless individuals and couples achieve their dream of conceiving a child. This procedure involves combining eggs and sperm outside of the body in a laboratory setting, and then transferring the resulting embryo(s) into the uterus for implantation.

The process of IVF begins with ovarian stimulation, where medications are administered to stimulate the ovaries to produce multiple eggs. These eggs are then retrieved through a minor surgical procedure and combined with sperm in a laboratory dish. The fertilized eggs, now embryos, are closely monitored for a few days to ensure their development.

Once the embryos have reached a certain stage of development, they are transferred into the uterus through a thin catheter. This procedure is relatively painless and does not require anesthesia. Following the embryo transfer, individuals or couples may need to take progesterone supplements to support the lining of the uterus and increase the chances of successful implantation.

It is important to note that the success rates of IVF can vary depending on various factors, including the age of the woman, the quality of the eggs and sperm, and any underlying fertility issues. Some individuals or couples may require multiple IVF cycles to achieve a successful pregnancy.

IVF has revolutionized the field of reproductive medicine and has provided hope to those struggling with infertility. It offers a viable option for individuals or couples who may have difficulty conceiving naturally due to factors such as blocked fallopian tubes, low sperm count, or unexplained infertility.

While IVF can be an emotionally and physically demanding process, the potential rewards of a successful pregnancy make it a popular choice for many. It is important to consult with a fertility specialist to determine if IVF is the right option for you and to discuss any potential risks or side effects associated with the procedure.

Intrauterine Insemination (IUI)

Intrauterine Insemination (IUI)

Intrauterine insemination (IUI) is a fertility treatment that involves placing sperm directly into a woman's uterus to increase the chances of conception. This procedure is commonly used for couples who are struggling with infertility or for individuals who are using donor sperm.

The process of IUI begins with the collection of sperm, either from the male partner or a sperm donor. The sperm is then washed and prepared in a laboratory to separate the healthy and motile sperm from the semen. This ensures that only the most viable sperm are used for the procedure.

During the actual IUI procedure, a thin catheter is inserted through the cervix and into the uterus. The prepared sperm sample is then injected into the uterus, bypassing the cervix and increasing the chances of the sperm reaching the fallopian tubes where fertilization can occur.

IUI is often used in conjunction with fertility medications to stimulate the ovaries and increase the number of eggs produced during a cycle. This helps to further enhance the chances of conception. The procedure itself is relatively quick and painless, with minimal discomfort experienced by the woman.

IUI can be an effective treatment option for couples with certain fertility issues, such as low sperm count or motility, mild endometriosis, or unexplained infertility. It offers a less invasive and more affordable alternative to more complex fertility treatments like in vitro fertilization (IVF).

However, it is important to note that the success rates of IUI can vary depending on various factors, including the age of the woman, the quality of the sperm, and the underlying cause of infertility. It may take multiple cycles of IUI before achieving a successful pregnancy.

Before undergoing IUI, it is recommended to consult with a fertility specialist who can assess your individual situation and provide guidance on the most appropriate treatment options. They can also discuss the potential risks and side effects associated with IUI, such as the possibility of multiple pregnancies.

In conclusion, intrauterine insemination (IUI) is a procedure that can help couples and individuals struggling with infertility to increase their chances of conception. By placing prepared sperm directly into the uterus, IUI bypasses potential barriers and improves the likelihood of fertilization. While it may not be suitable for everyone, IUI offers a less invasive and more affordable option compared to other fertility treatments. If you are considering IUI, it is important to consult with a fertility specialist who can provide personalized advice and guidance.

Egg Freezing

Egg freezing, also known as oocyte cryopreservation, is a revolutionary technique that allows women to preserve their fertility by freezing their eggs for future use. This process involves the extraction of a woman's eggs, which are then carefully frozen and stored until she is ready to use them for conception.

There are several reasons why women may choose to freeze their eggs. One common scenario is when a woman wants to delay starting a family due to career or personal reasons. By freezing her eggs at a younger age when they are at their peak quality, she can increase her chances of successful conception later in life when she is ready to have a child.

Egg freezing is also beneficial for women who are facing medical treatments that may potentially harm their fertility, such as chemotherapy or radiation therapy. By freezing their eggs before undergoing these treatments, they can preserve their ability to have biological children in the future.

Another advantage of egg freezing is that it allows women to take control of their reproductive timeline. It provides a sense of security and peace of mind, knowing that their eggs are safely stored and available whenever they are ready to start a family. It can alleviate the pressure and anxiety associated with the biological clock, giving women more flexibility and options when it comes to family planning.

The process of egg freezing involves several steps. First, a woman undergoes ovarian stimulation, where she takes hormonal medications to stimulate the ovaries to produce multiple eggs. This is followed by regular monitoring through ultrasound scans and blood tests to determine the optimal time for egg retrieval.

The actual egg retrieval procedure is performed under sedation and involves the insertion of a thin needle into the ovaries to collect the mature eggs. The collected eggs are then carefully frozen using a technique called vitrification, which ensures their preservation and quality.

When a woman decides to use her frozen eggs, they are thawed and fertilized with sperm through a process called in vitro fertilization (IVF). The resulting embryos are then transferred to the woman's uterus for potential implantation and pregnancy.

Egg freezing has opened up new possibilities for women to take control of their reproductive choices and preserve their fertility. It offers a sense of empowerment and flexibility, allowing women to pursue their goals and dreams without the worry of a ticking biological clock. With advances in technology and increasing success rates, egg freezing continues to provide hope and options for women who want to preserve their fertility for the future.

Common Fertility Problems

Common fertility problems can greatly hinder the conception process for individuals or couples trying to conceive. It is important to identify and understand these common issues in order to seek appropriate treatment and increase the chances of successful conception. Here are some of the most prevalent fertility problems:

- **Polycystic Ovary Syndrome (PCOS):** PCOS is a hormonal disorder that affects women of reproductive age. It can cause irregular menstrual cycles, hormonal imbalances, and the formation of cysts on the ovaries. PCOS can make it difficult for women to ovulate regularly, hindering their chances of conception.
- **Endometriosis:** Endometriosis is a condition in which the tissue that normally lines the uterus

grows outside of it. This can lead to inflammation, scar tissue formation, and the development of ovarian cysts. Endometriosis can affect fertility by causing blockages in the fallopian tubes or affecting the quality of eggs.
- **Male Infertility:** Male infertility is often caused by issues with sperm production, sperm motility, or sperm health. Common causes include low sperm count, poor sperm quality, or blockages in the reproductive tract. Male infertility can significantly reduce the chances of successful fertilization.

Identifying these common fertility problems is the first step towards finding appropriate solutions. It is important to consult with a healthcare professional specializing in fertility to diagnose the specific issues and develop a personalized treatment plan. With the right interventions and support, many fertility problems can be overcome, leading to successful conception and the fulfillment of the desire to have a child.

Polycystic Ovary Syndrome (PCOS)

Polycystic Ovary Syndrome (PCOS) is a common hormonal disorder that affects women of reproductive age. It is characterized by the presence of multiple cysts on the ovaries, irregular menstrual cycles, and high levels of androgens (male hormones) in the body. PCOS can have a significant impact on fertility, making it difficult for women with the condition to conceive.

One of the main challenges for women with PCOS is irregular ovulation or the absence of ovulation altogether. Ovulation is the process in which an egg is released from the ovary and is necessary for fertilization to occur. Without regular ovulation, the chances of getting pregnant naturally are greatly reduced.

Fortunately, there are treatment options available for women with PCOS who are trying to conceive. One common approach is the use of medications such as clomiphene citrate, which helps stimulate ovulation. This medication works by blocking the effects of estrogen in the body, which in turn stimulates the release of follicle-stimulating hormone (FSH) from the pituitary gland. FSH then stimulates the growth and development of ovarian follicles, leading to ovulation.

In addition to medication, lifestyle changes can also play a significant role in managing PCOS and improving fertility. Maintaining a healthy weight through regular exercise and a balanced diet can help regulate hormone levels and promote regular ovulation. It is important to focus on consuming whole foods, such as fruits, vegetables, lean proteins, and whole grains, while limiting processed foods and refined sugars.

Furthermore, managing stress levels and practicing stress-reducing techniques, such as yoga or meditation, can also have a positive impact on fertility in women with PCOS.

Stress can disrupt hormone balance and interfere with ovulation, so finding effective ways to relax and unwind is crucial.

In some cases, assisted reproductive technologies may be necessary for women with PCOS who are struggling to conceive. These include procedures such as in vitro fertilization (IVF) or intrauterine insemination (IUI), which can help bypass ovulation issues and increase the chances of successful pregnancy.

Overall, while PCOS can present challenges when it comes to fertility, there are various treatment options and lifestyle changes that can help improve the chances of conception. It is important for women with PCOS to work closely with their healthcare providers to develop a personalized treatment plan that addresses their specific needs and goals.

Endometriosis

Endometriosis:

Endometriosis is a common condition that affects many women and can have a significant impact on fertility. It occurs when the tissue that lines the uterus, known as the endometrium, grows outside of the uterus. This tissue can attach itself to various organs in the pelvic area, such as the ovaries, fallopian tubes, and the lining of the pelvis.

When a woman with endometriosis ovulates, the endometrial tissue outside the uterus also responds to hormonal changes, causing it to thicken and break down, just like the tissue inside the uterus. However, unlike the tissue inside the uterus, the blood and tissue shed from the endometrial implants have no way to exit the body. This can lead to the formation of scar tissue, adhesions, and the development of cysts called endometriomas.

The presence of endometriosis can significantly impact fertility. The scar tissue and adhesions can cause organs to stick together, affecting the normal functioning of the reproductive system. In severe cases, the fallopian tubes may become blocked or distorted, making it difficult for the egg to travel from the ovaries to the uterus. Additionally, the inflammatory response caused by endometriosis can interfere with the release of eggs and the implantation of a fertilized egg in the uterus.

Fortunately, there are treatment options available for women with endometriosis who are trying to conceive. Depending on the severity of the condition and the individual's goals, treatment may involve medication to manage symptoms, surgery to remove endometrial implants and scar tissue, or assisted reproductive technologies such as in vitro fertilization (IVF).

It is important for women with endometriosis who are trying to conceive to consult with a healthcare professional specializing in reproductive medicine. They can provide personalized advice and guidance on the best treatment options based on individual circumstances. By addressing the effects of endometriosis on fertility, women can increase their chances of successfully conceiving and starting a family.

Male Infertility

Male infertility is a common issue that can hinder the process of conception. There are various factors that can contribute to male infertility, ranging from medical conditions to lifestyle choices. Understanding these causes is crucial in order to identify potential solutions and increase the chances of successful conception.

One of the main causes of male infertility is low sperm count or poor sperm quality. This can be attributed to factors such as hormonal imbalances, genetic disorders, or certain medical conditions like varicocele. Additionally, lifestyle choices like smoking, excessive alcohol consumption, and drug use can also have a negative impact on sperm production and quality.

Another common cause of male infertility is abnormal sperm function or motility. Sperm motility refers to the ability of sperm to move and swim effectively towards the egg for fertilization. Issues with sperm motility can be caused by genetic factors, infections, or hormonal imbalances. Poor sperm motility can significantly reduce the chances of successful fertilization.

Fortunately, there are potential solutions available for male infertility. In some cases, medical treatments such as hormone therapy or surgery can help address the underlying causes of infertility. Lifestyle changes, such as quitting smoking, reducing alcohol consumption, and maintaining a healthy weight, can also improve sperm production and quality.

Furthermore, assisted reproductive technologies like in vitro fertilization (IVF) and intracytoplasmic sperm injection (ICSI) can be utilized to overcome male infertility. These procedures involve the retrieval of sperm and the direct injection of a single sperm into the egg, increasing the chances of successful fertilization.

In conclusion, male infertility can be caused by a variety of factors, including low sperm count, poor sperm quality, and abnormal sperm function. Identifying the underlying causes is essential in order to explore potential solutions and increase the chances of successful conception. Medical treatments, lifestyle changes, and assisted reproductive technologies can all play a role in addressing male infertility and helping individuals or couples achieve their goal of starting a family.

Optimizing Fertility

Optimizing fertility is a crucial step for individuals or couples who are trying to conceive. By following certain tips and advice, you can increase the chances of successful conception and fulfill your dream of starting a family. Here are some key strategies to optimize fertility:

- **Maintain a Healthy Lifestyle:** A healthy lifestyle plays a significant role in promoting fertility. Make sure to eat a balanced diet rich in fruits, vegetables, whole grains, and lean proteins. Regular exercise can also improve fertility by reducing stress and maintaining a healthy weight.

- **Understand Timing and Frequency:** Timing intercourse correctly is essential for maximizing the chances of conception. Tracking your menstrual cycle and identifying the fertile window can help you determine the best time to try for a baby. Aim for regular intercourse every 2-3 days throughout the month to increase the likelihood of sperm meeting the egg.
- **Manage Stress:** Stress can have a negative impact on fertility. Find effective stress management techniques that work for you, such as yoga, meditation, or engaging in hobbies you enjoy. Taking time to relax and unwind can help create a more favorable environment for conception.

Additionally, it's important to avoid smoking, excessive alcohol consumption, and exposure to environmental toxins, as these factors can significantly reduce fertility. It's also advisable to limit caffeine intake and consult with a healthcare professional about any medications you may be taking that could affect fertility.

Remember, optimizing fertility is a process that requires patience and dedication. By implementing these strategies and seeking guidance from a healthcare provider, you can increase your chances of successful conception and embark on the journey of parenthood.

Healthy Lifestyle

A healthy lifestyle plays a crucial role in promoting fertility. It is important to maintain a balanced diet and engage in regular exercise to optimize your chances of conceiving. Here are some key factors to consider when it comes to a healthy lifestyle and fertility:

- **Diet:** A nutritious diet is essential for reproductive health. Include a variety of fruits, vegetables, whole grains, lean proteins, and healthy fats in your meals. Certain foods, such as leafy greens, berries, nuts, and seeds, are rich in antioxidants and can support fertility. It is also advisable to limit your intake of processed foods, sugary snacks, and beverages.
- **Exercise:** Regular physical activity can help regulate hormone levels, improve blood circulation, and maintain a healthy weight, all of which contribute to fertility. Engage in moderate exercise, such as brisk walking, swimming, or cycling, for at least 30 minutes most days of the week. However, avoid excessive exercise as it can negatively impact fertility.
- **Weight Management:** Maintaining a healthy weight is crucial for fertility. Both being overweight and underweight can affect hormone production and disrupt the menstrual cycle. If you are overweight, losing a moderate amount

of weight can improve your chances of conceiving. Conversely, if you are underweight, gaining some weight may help regulate your menstrual cycle.

- **Hydration:** Staying adequately hydrated is important for overall health and fertility. Drink plenty of water throughout the day to support the production of cervical mucus, which aids in sperm transport and fertilization.
- **Limit Alcohol and Caffeine:** Excessive alcohol and caffeine consumption can negatively impact fertility. It is advisable to limit your intake of alcoholic beverages and caffeinated drinks, such as coffee and soda, when trying to conceive.
- **Manage Stress:** High levels of stress can interfere with hormonal balance and ovulation. Find healthy ways to manage stress, such as practicing relaxation techniques, exercising, or engaging in hobbies you enjoy.

Remember, a healthy lifestyle is not only beneficial for fertility but also for your overall well-being. By adopting these habits, you are taking proactive steps towards optimizing your chances of successful conception.

Timing and Frequency

The timing and frequency of intercourse play a crucial role in maximizing the chances of conception. Understanding the menstrual cycle and identifying the fertile window are key factors in determining the optimal timing for intercourse.

During a woman's menstrual cycle, there are specific days when she is most fertile and likely to conceive. This fertile window typically occurs around the time of ovulation, which is when an egg is released from the ovary. Ovulation usually takes place around the middle of the menstrual cycle, approximately 14 days before the start of the next period.

To increase the chances of conception, it is recommended to have intercourse regularly during the fertile window. Sperm can survive in the female reproductive system for up to five days, so having intercourse a few days before ovulation and on the day of ovulation itself can greatly enhance the likelihood of fertilization.

Tracking ovulation can be done through various methods, such as monitoring changes in cervical mucus or using ovulation predictor kits. These tools can help pinpoint the most fertile days and guide couples in timing intercourse for optimal results.

It is important to note that stress and pressure to conceive can negatively impact fertility. Therefore, it is essential for couples to approach the process with a relaxed and positive mindset. Enjoying intimacy and maintaining a healthy relationship can contribute to a more conducive environment for conception.

Additionally, it is worth mentioning that frequency of intercourse can also affect fertility. While it is generally recommended to have intercourse every two to three days throughout the menstrual cycle, excessive or too frequent intercourse may reduce sperm count and motility. It is important to strike a balance and maintain a moderate frequency to ensure the best chances of conception.

In summary, understanding the optimal timing and frequency of intercourse is crucial for maximizing the chances of conception. Identifying the fertile window, having regular intercourse during this period, and maintaining a relaxed and positive mindset can greatly enhance fertility and increase the likelihood of successful conception.

Stress Management

Stress can have a significant impact on fertility and the ability to conceive. When the body is under stress, it releases stress hormones such as cortisol, which can disrupt the delicate hormonal balance necessary for ovulation and fertilization. High levels of stress can also affect the quality and motility of sperm, making it more difficult for fertilization to occur.

Fortunately, there are techniques that can help manage and reduce stress during the conception process. One effective method is practicing relaxation techniques such as deep breathing, meditation, and yoga. These activities can help calm the mind and body, reducing stress levels and promoting a more favorable environment for conception.

In addition to relaxation techniques, maintaining a healthy lifestyle can also play a crucial role in managing stress. Regular exercise, a balanced diet, and adequate sleep can all contribute to overall well-being and stress reduction. It is also important to make time for self-care activities that bring joy and relaxation, such as reading, spending time with loved ones, or engaging in hobbies.

Another helpful strategy for managing stress during the conception process is seeking support from others. Talking to a trusted friend, family member, or therapist can provide a safe space to express emotions, fears, and concerns. Support groups or online communities can also offer a sense of connection and understanding during this challenging time.

It is important to remember that managing stress is a personal journey, and what works for one person may not work for another. It may take some trial and error to find the techniques that are most effective in reducing stress and promoting fertility. However, by prioritizing stress management and taking steps to create a more relaxed and balanced lifestyle, individuals and couples can increase their chances of successful conception.

Frequently Asked Questions

- **What is ovulation and why is it important for getting pregnant?**

  Ovulation is the release of an egg from the ovary, which occurs once a month in women of reproductive age. It is a crucial step in the conception process because fertilization can only occur if sperm meets the egg during this fertile period.

- **How can I track my ovulation?**

There are several methods to track ovulation, including monitoring changes in basal body temperature, observing changes in cervical mucus, using ovulation predictor kits, or tracking menstrual cycles. These methods can help you identify your most fertile days and increase your chances of getting pregnant.

- **What factors can affect sperm viability?**

Sperm viability can be influenced by various factors such as age, overall health, lifestyle choices, and exposure to certain environmental factors. It is important to maintain a healthy lifestyle, avoid excessive alcohol consumption, quit smoking, and minimize exposure to toxins to improve sperm viability.

- **How long does sperm survive inside the female reproductive system?**

Sperm can typically survive inside the female reproductive system for up to five days. However, the chances of fertilization are highest within the first two to three days after intercourse.

- **What can I do to improve sperm motility?**

Healthy lifestyle choices, such as regular exercise, a balanced diet, and reducing stress levels, can contribute to improved sperm motility. Additionally, avoiding excessive heat exposure, such as hot baths or saunas, can also help maintain optimal sperm motility.

- **How does age affect fertility?**

Age plays a significant role in fertility, especially for women. As women age, the number and quality of their eggs decline, making it more challenging to conceive. Men also experience a decline in fertility with age, although the impact is generally less pronounced compared to women.

- **What are some common health conditions that can affect fertility?**

Health conditions such as polycystic ovary syndrome (PCOS), endometriosis, and certain sexually transmitted infections can affect fertility. It is important to seek medical advice if you suspect any underlying health conditions that may be impacting your ability to conceive.

- **What are assisted reproductive technologies?**

Assisted reproductive technologies (ART) are medical procedures or treatments that assist individuals or couples in achieving pregnancy. Examples include in vitro fertilization (IVF), intrauterine insemination (IUI), and egg freezing. These techniques are often recommended for those struggling with infertility.

- **What are some common fertility problems?**

Common fertility problems include conditions such as polycystic ovary syndrome (PCOS), endometriosis, and male infertility issues. These conditions can make it more difficult to conceive and may require medical intervention or treatment.

- **How can I optimize my fertility?**

To optimize fertility, it is important to maintain a healthy lifestyle, including a nutritious diet, regular exercise, and stress management techniques. Understanding your menstrual cycle and timing intercourse during the fertile window can also increase your chances of successful conception.

Have Questions / Comments?

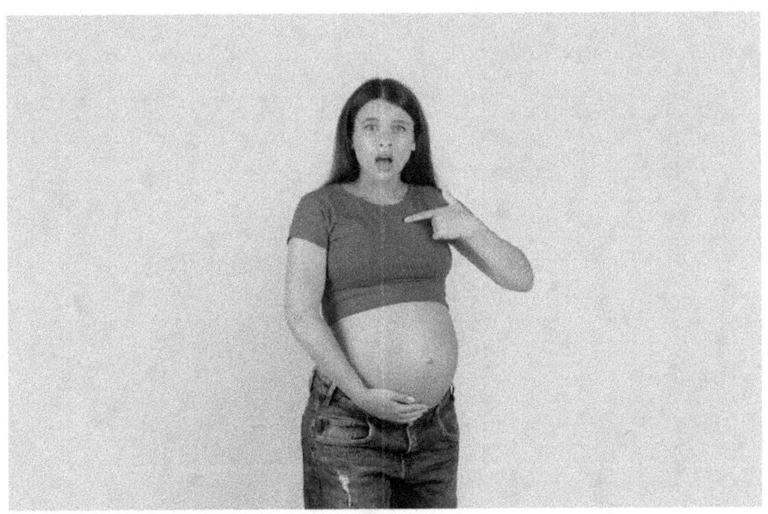

This book was designed to cover as much info as possible but I know I have probably missed something, or some new amazing discovery that has just come out.

If you notice something missing or have a question that I failed to answer, please get in touch and let me know. If I can, I will email you an answer and also update the book so others can also benefit from it.

Thanks For Being Awesome :)

Submit Your Questions / Comments At:

Get How To Be A Super Mom - 100% FREE

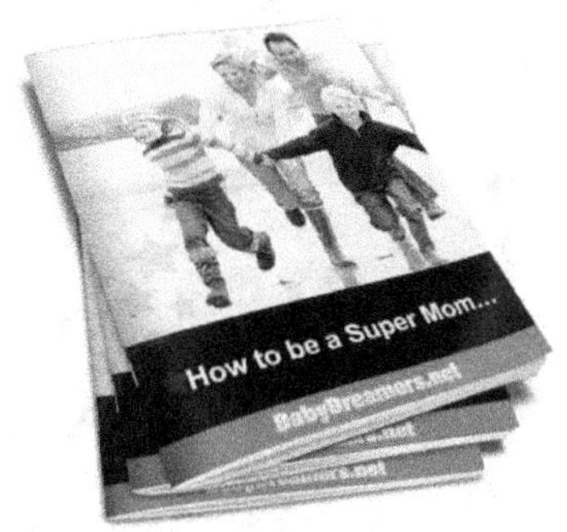

For being one of our amazing readers, we would love to offer you another book we have created, 100% free.

Being a mom is probably the most important job in the world – we've all heard that, and it's true. You're bringing up the next generation of wonderful, intelligent, loving, creative, responsible people.

We all want to be Super Mom and to be everything and do everything, but it this possible?

Being a Super Mom is possible, but you have to learn how to empower yourself to be the kind of Super Mom that you feel you need to be, keeping in mind that the title Super Mom doesn't mean the same thing to everyone.

Get How to be a Super Mom For Free at

BabyDreamers.net